KETO DIET 1X1

The Guide to Rapid Weight Loss - Fast and Easy Recipes for Every Day incl. 21 Days Weight Loss Plan

MATTHEW JOSH

TABLE OF CONTENTS

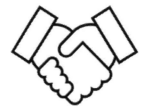

Welcome to a world where cauliflower becomes grains of rice and pizza bases.

A world of breadless burger buns, courgette lasagne sheets and lettuce tortillas.

A world of fat-packed, oil dripping, finger-licking, whole-hearted goodness.

Because in this world you don't have to hold back.

In this world, you can gnaw on a block of cheese and feel good about it.

You can crack an entire 12-pack of eggs into a pan, scramble them up and gobble them all down knowing that your body is absolutely loving it.

You can drench your desserts in an ocean of double cream, lose your lunch in a sea of mayonnaise, bury your breakfast in a trench of peanut butter, knowing that none of it will turn into body fat. Instead, the fat that you eat becomes your main source of energy. And in this world, you are going to have plenty more of that.

How? Why? We'll get to that.

Welcome to the world of keto.

INTRODUCTION

In this book, we will walk you through the necessary learning process that can lead you to becoming a fat-burning machine.

To begin with we will introduce you to keto, teach you about what it is, how it functions, and how it can transform your life. We will explore the science behind it, before we teach you how to keto. Here you will learn the dos and don'ts of the keto diet and how to manage your intake of carbohydrates, fibre, fat and protein in order to maximise keto's bountiful benefits.

And then, once you have the understanding, we will throw a wealth of delicious recipes at you to help you become fully accomplished in the art of living the keto-lifestyle. We will give you everything, from tasty pasta and rice alternatives to the fanciest, most flamboyant keto dishes.

First and foremost, let us kick you off with a brief explanation of what you're getting yourself into. I recommend cementing this in your brain, as I can guarantee you people are going to question your choice to go keto. The Keto diet is a diet which involves restricting our intake of carbohydrates and sugars and instead, increasing our intake of fat. When we eat carbohydrates and sugar, the body turns them into glucose, which we run off for energy. So, if we significantly decrease our intake of these foods, then the body turns to another source of energy. Fat. When our systems are so high in glucose, the fat that we eat stores in the body. But when stop eating so much glucose, we run off fat as our energy and we burn it relentlessly. This state is referred to as ketosis. This results in a drastic shedding of body fat, as well as multiple other benefits which we will explain later on. But, long story short, cut the sugary foods and bring on the fatty ones.

If you have already heard mentioning's of the keto diet, you may perhaps have a perception of it as boring, restricting, or even limiting. We can't deny, some of your favourite things will have to go, therefore, you could say it is restricting. There may be circumstances where you're at the train station, and there are only carb-crammed sandwiches and sugar-fuelled drinks on offer. In that regard, it can be seen as limiting.

But boring? No way. Okay, so we may have to give up a few things. But what goes can be replaced, and this opens a doorway to a world of food combinations and creations that you've probably never even imagined. Yes, there may be certain occasions when it's a bit harder to be spontaneous when out and about. But we adapt. We learn to become more organized with our food. Learn what we can snack on. This sounds like we have to become really responsible and disciplined. That's a great attribute to learn for sure, and getting into keto will help with that for sure. But as you become more familiar with the keto ways, you learn how to become more flexible and you start to learn what you can get away with. Just wait until you're a few weeks in to the low-carb lifestyle and you're eating cheese directly from the block. Just wait until you walk out of a newsagents armed with a bag of nuts and a jar of olives, ready to snack until your jaw starts to hurt. Just wait until you smother a jar of blueberries in peanut butter and endless amounts of double cream. Because don't forget – while the door closes on carbs and sugar, the doorway to fat has swung wide open.

So, enough with the romanticism. Let's talk facts.

WHAT IS THE KETO DIET?

THE SCIENCE

Eat more fat, carry less fat. How can that possibly work? Basically, the body can run on two different fuels. Glucose (sugar) and fat. As we briefly explained in the intro, when we eat large amounts of carbohydrates, they turn into glucose and we run off that for energy. This means that the majority of the fat that we eat is stored rather than using it for fuel. The keto diet means that we eat a diet so low in carbs that we switch to using mainly fat for fuel. Even the brain can become fuelled by fat. When the body is out of sugar, fat is converted in the liver into energy molecules called ketones that fuel the brain. The diet that results in this is called the ketogenic diet, shorten ketogenic, and alas, we have the keto diet.

Benefits

Ketosis is the name given to the state when the body is fuelled mostly by fat. One major benefit that draws many people to the keto diet is that you burn fat 24-7, including while you sleep. This ease of fat burning is aided by a significant drop in insulin (the fat-storing hormone) levels without increased hunger.

Some people use the keto diet specifically to improve their mental performance, while it is extremely common for people to experience increased energy levels when in ketosis. Due to improving your body's ability to access its fat stores, people often experience vastly increased physical endurance. When we are running off stored carbohydrates (glucose), this only supplies us with a couple of hours of intense exercise, or less. But your fat stores carry enough energy that can potentially last weeks. Much more visibly, the vast reduction in body-fat weight will be a valuable improvement in many competitive sports, including endurance sports.

It is very common for people to feel a dramatic increase in their appetite control, while feelings of hunger decrease significantly, making it easier to eat less and lose excess weight. This distinct lack of hunger makes it easier to carry out intermittent fasting which is widely proven to speed up weight loss, enhance efforts to reverse type 2 diabetes beyond just ketos effects. As the ketogenic diet itself reduces blood-sugar levels, the need for medications and reduces the potentially damaging impact of high insulin levels, it makes complete sense that not only efforts to reverse type-2 diabetes are aided by the ketogenic diet, it aids in prevention of getting the disease as well.

Meanwhile, the keto diet can lead to a calmer stomach, where people experience less gas, fewer cramps, less pain and feeling less bloated after meals. This can often result in improvements in IBS symptoms. A keto diet can also help treat high blood pressure, result in less acne and help those who suffer with migraine symptoms. It may also help with epilepsy, PCOS, heartburn, reduce sugar cravings and help combat mental health issues alongside many other potential benefits.

Risks and Drawbacks

While this diet can and has proven to have transformative effects on people's lives, it is important to consider that it may not be for you. We will explore potential side effects and discuss potential risks later in "how do I know if I'm in ketosis?" section, where we will consider if the keto diet is right for you.

The keto diet is very similar to many other fad diets that have trended in the past, such as the Poleo diet, gluten-free diets and, in particular, the Atkins diet. What is different with keto is that it is a supercharged low carb diet where you make sure that you experience the maximum benefits.

HOW TO KETO

So, what's the deal? What can I eat? And how much? What can't I eat? And what if I break the rules?

Let's get down to it.

GETTING INTO KETOSIS

Particularly at the beginning of your keto journey, it's important to gather an understanding of how to measure your net-carb intake. It's pretty straight forward - fibre counteracts carbs, so net-carbs are the carbohydrate content that a food contains, minus its fibre content. Yes, it's true; particularly during the early stages of your transition to keto, you're going to have to become a label reader.

There are different ways you can eat a low carb diet. You can take the liberal route, which is where you aim for a net carb intake of 50-100 grams per day. It is unlikely you will enter a full state of ketosis like this, but you will likely lose fat a bit easier as the body has less glucose to burn before it accesses the fat.

You can take the moderate route, of 25-50 grams of carbs per day. This will greatly increase your chances of entering ketosis.

But a ketogenic diet means eating 0-25 grams of carbs per day. Sticking to this consistently will enter you into a state of ketosis.

We have some pointers that will help you get there without straying from the track.

1. **First and foremost, Reduce your carb intake.** You'll get good at checking the label for carb content, and subtracting the fibre away from it to work out if the food you're wondering about is suitable for a keto diet. And as time wears on, you'll have to check the label less and less as you learn what works and what doesn't.

2. **Ensure you eat enough fat.** The beauty of the keto diet is that you can now pile in the fat. Fat supplies your energy, so make sure you are getting enough of it. Roll in mayo, shower in butter. Also eat plenty of protein and low carb veggies and you'll be golden.

3. **While eating enough protein is important, it is key to not eat too much of it.** We recommend 1.2-2g of protein per kg of reference body weight per day. So, for example, if I weigh 80kg, I would eat 96-160g of protein per day. This is because amino acids from protein foods can be converted to glucose, but that is very rare. Nonetheless, better to stay on the safe side and keep on track to ketosis.

4. **Avoiding snacking and adding intermittent fasting** will aid your path to ketosis too.

5. **Exercise.** Exercise is always important. Any kind of exercise on a low carb diet can moderately increase your ketone levels.

6. **Manage your sleep and stress levels.** Sleep deprivation and stress hormones raise blood sugar levels, slowing ketosis and weight loss.

7. **Supplements are not required for the keto diet.** There are some you can buy, but it is not necessary for getting to ketosis.

How do I know I'm in Ketosis?

While there are official things that you can do to measure it, such as urine tests, blood and breath samples there are tell-tale signs that the process is beginning. They aren't all that great though, to be frank.

Now, it's important to acknowledge that the transition off your energy source can have some interesting effects on your body. When you suddenly switch your body's metabolism from burning glucose to fat and ketones, you may experience some side effects as your body adapts – especially between days two and five.

These effects may include a headache, tiredness, muscle fatigue, cramping and heart palpitations. They are typically short term, and there are ways to minimise or cure them. To reduce potential side effects, you may decide to gradually decrease your consumption of carbs over a few weeks, but like this the results will come slower, of course. Experiencing these side effects is regarded as the keto flu, and the symptoms will often disappear within a week or two as your body adapts to increased fat burning. Eating carbs tends to result in swelling (excess water retention) within the body, which isn't great for us. So, when you start a low carb diet you may notice that this excess fluid is lost and that you urinate more, and with that some extra salt is lost too. The result of this is dehydration and a lack of salt which appear to be the two major causes of the keto flu. I'm sure you can imagine how they are solved. Drink more water than usual, and increase your salt intake. Tasty ways to increase your salt intake include drinking a cup of bouillon or broth once or twice a day. You can also simply spoon salt into a glass of water – but we appreciate that that may not be for everybody.

Once you move beyond this stage though, you should start to feel an increase of energy levels. To accompany this, many people experience reduced hunger. In fact, many people find themselves just wanting to eat once or twice a day – doing some form of intermittent fasting, which really helps with the process of entering ketosis.

WHAT TO EAT

Right then. We've looked at the science, we know what's happening in the body. Now for the juicy part. What can I eat, what can't I eat? Sacrifices must be made, but don't worry, there are plenty of positives in here too as certain foods that you may have previously believed to be "bad" for you because they are full of fat become superfoods.

Green Light

Meat – We'll always advise you to choose organic and grass-fed meat. Not just because it's better for the environment and the creatures themselves, but because it's healthier and tastier that way too. Beef, pork, lamb, game and poultry all contain minimal carbs and the best part is that you don't need to hold back on eating the super tasty high-fat parts, such as the skin on the chicken and the crackling from the pork.

Fish and seafood – All great. High fat, high protein, minimal carbs. Again, seeking local, fresh fish is typically going to taste better and have a healthier impact on your body and the environment.

Eggs – Organic is always the way, but all kinds of eggs are brilliant fuel for a keto diet.

Natural fats such as butter, cream and oil make food taste better. You no longer need to hold back on them and in fact we encourage the opposite. Go wild.

Vegetables – Now this is where it gets interesting. All kinds of vegetables that grow above ground, such as lettuce, broccoli, courgette, olives, spinach, mushrooms, peppers and tomatoes are absolute essentials in this diet. However, you will see later that not all vegetables are suitable for keto.

Dairy products – Always select the full-fat options. Real butter, cream, cheese, yoghurt. Lap it up.

Nuts and berries – low carb nuts like brazil nuts, macadamias and almonds are great. Raspberries, strawberries and blueberries are good but in moderation.

Drinks – Now. Alcohol. This is where some people may have to make some life changes. Red wine drinkers, you're in the clear, but moderate. Straight spirit drinkers, you're in there too. Soft drinks wise – teas and coffees are the best, and of course lots and lots of water.

Red Light

Sugar – Fizzy drinks, fruit juices, cakes, buns, pastries, ice cream, breakfast cereals. See ya. But there are low carb, low sugar alternatives for some of these that will blow your mind.

Starch – Bread, pasta, rice, potatoes. Don't panic, we have alternatives in this very book.

Root vegetables – So vegetables that below the ground, such as carrots and potatoes tend to be very high in carbs, but you *can* include *some* in a very moderated way.

Beer – Oh beer. Sweet, sweet, heavenly beer. To be honest, giving up beer wasn't as bad as I'd have thought. Hangover's are easier as you feel significantly less heavier, and I now drastically prefer the vast variety offered by wines.

Fruit – so yes – a lot of fruit actually leaves the menu too. This is the most surprising bit for most people. Many fruits are high in carbs and sugar. It's like nature's candy. Treat it like that. Evolutionarily, we would only have eaten fruit as a rare treat on the occasions someone ventured to fetch it. When you really feel like treating yourself, have a piece of fruit. I can almost guarantee that you will appreciate the flavour more.

Special Occasions

- Dry white wine in small doses

- Dark chocolate above 70% cocoa

So, that's it. You're bursting with knowledge and have gathered an understanding of what you can and can't eat to get into ketosis. You're ready to start your ketogenic diet.

THE KETO BASICS

HOW TO REPLACE BREAD, RICE, PASTA AND, MOST IMPORTANTLY, PIZZA

Here we're going to give you the basic tips you need to flourish as a keto master. None of us want to lose the taste, texture and general sustenance that pasta, rice and bread provide in our lives, surely? Well, we don't have to, and below we will explain how to substitute these foods.

Basic Substitutions

Right, so everything with keto sounds great so far. More energy. More focus. More tasty food to add to your repertoire. The science is backed and straight forward enough to explain to your friends when they inevitably question why you don't want to get a fast-food takeaway.

But let's not overlook one pulsating fear all that all keto newcomers carry; "How can I possibly move on from rice, bread and pasta?"

We're not going to hide from the fact that many of the world's most delectable cuisines consist of these high-carb foods. So how about instead of giving them up, we find ways to replace them with health-packed, flavour-filled, low-carb versions.

RICE

Let's cut to the chase, here. Stick cauliflower in a blender. You have cauliflower rice. Simple as that. Don't have a blender? Get a decent cheese grater. Or you can even just savagely rip it to shreds using a knife. Both are a bit messy, but it works a treat and the important thing is that you end up with a rice-like consistency that tastes good. You can do the same with Broccoli, cabbage - even carrot if you like. And there you have it. A few lines of reading and I bet for some of you, that's a mind-blowing revelation that you've never considered. I don't even need to tell you the science behind it; swapping wheat for vegetables is inevitably going to be good for you.

And of course, you can do just as many variations of these kinds of rice as you would see on your standard Indian takeaway menu. Egg-fried. Coconut rice. Pilau.

But most importantly, you can make a beautiful risotto. And that is what we're going to teach you.

MUSHROOM CAULIFLOWER RICE RISOTTO

INGREDIENTS (FOR 2 SERVINGS):

- 1 tablespoon coconut oil
- 100g mushrooms
- 200g cauliflower, riced
- 100ml coconut cream
- 1 tablespoon nutritional yeast
- 2 leaves parsley

METHOD:

1   Melt coconut oil in a large pan before adding garlic and cooking until slightly golden.
2   Add the mushrooms and sauté for about 4-5 until tender and lightly browned.
3   Add in your pre-riced cauliflower (use a blender, cheese grater or a knife to rice your cauliflower) and stir until well blended with the mushrooms.
4   Stir in the coconut cream and nutritional yeast until heated. Remove from the heat, sling on the parsley garnish and you're good to go.

BREAD

Burger buns. Crackers. Sandwiches. Toast. It's not time to say goodbye to bread. Nor should it ever be. You'd be shocked how easy it is to make some of these bread alternatives. Here, we're going to get you cracking with a beautiful keto-bread bun.

KETO BREAD BUNS

INGREDIENTS (FOR 6 SERVINGS):

- 1/3 cup ground psyllium husk powder
- 3 egg whites
- 2 teaspoons baking powder
- 1¼ cups almond flour
- 1 cup water
- 2 tablespoon sesame seeds (optional)
- 2 teaspoon cider vinegar
- 1 teaspoon sea salt

METHOD:

1 Preheat the oven to 175c.

2 Combine the dry ingredients together and mix them in while you bring water to the boil.

3 Add the vinegar and egg whites to the dry mixture. Mix them until they are well introduced before slowly adding the boiling water while you beat the mixture with a hand mixer. Do this for about 30 seconds.

4 In order to not over mix the dough, aim for a consistency resembling play-doh. If you don't know what play-doh is, then I truly feel for you.

5 Moisten your hands with a little olive oil and shape the dough into 6 separate rolls before placing them on a greased baking sheet and topping with sesame seeds.

6 Bake on the lower rack of the over for 50-60 minutes (depending on the size of the rolls). Tap the bottom of the buns, and if they are hollow then you know that they are cooked. Don't undercook them. Not good.

7 I could give you serving tips, but it's bread; do with it as you please.

PASTA

If you love pasta, time to get creative. Bean pasta is blooming marvellous. I still can't quite wrap my head around how various beans can be strung into spaghetti, swivelled into penne or wrapped into ravioli. But it happens. It's certainly a thing. And you can buy them in most major supermarkets or online. Somewhere in the world, the keto guru's will be able to teach you the magic of how it is formed. But for now, we're simply going to give you a scrumptious recipe to combine with your bean spag.

KETO CARBONARA

Nutrition:

Net carbs – 5g
Protein – 20g
Fat – 53g
Calories – 586

INGREDIENTS (2 SERVINGS):

- 100g slender soy bean spaghetti
- 20g butter
- 4 rashers chopped bacon
- 1 clove minced garlic
- ½ cup cream
- 30g finely grated parmesan cheese
- Salt and pepper

METHOD:

1. Whilst bringing a large pot of water to the boil, place a frying pan on medium heat and add the butter and the bacon. Cook for 5-6 minutes until golden brown, stirring occasionally.
2. Once the water has come to the boil, add the spaghetti and cook for 3-5 minutes (until al dente).
3. Strain off the water and set aside whilst the sauce cooks.
4. Once the bacon is cooked, add the garlic for about 30 seconds without burning.
5. Turn to a low heat and add the cream to the bacon mixture, scraping the bottom of the pan to ensure you don't miss out on any of the crispy bacon bits.
6. Allow the sauce to simmer for 1-2 minutes until it thickens and then remove it from the heat. Season the sauce with salt and pepper.
7. Add the parmesan and the cooked spaghetti and then stir until the spaghetti is coated with the creamy sauce. Top with extra grated parmesan and parsley and voila, low-carb carbonara.

PIZZA

Now, I'm fully aware that, technically, pizza would fall under the bread section. But I want you keto-newcomers to be clear, this is not the end of the road for pizza. In fact, with this new lifestyle, your pizzas are about to become even cheesier than ever – and you needn't carry even a smidgen of guilt about it! Here you will learn to make a delicious keto pizza which should only take about 30 minutes from the moment you step into the kitchen equipped with the ingredients.

KETO PIZZA

INGREDIENTS (FOR 1 PIZZA):

- 2 large eggs
- 2 tablespoon melted butter
- 2 tablespoon cottage cheese (sour cream can be substituted)
- 1 cup almond flour
- ½ teaspoon garlic powder
- ¼ teaspoon pink Himalayan or sea salt
- 1 cup shredded cheddar cheese
- Whatever toppings you desire (just ensure to acknowledge the net carbs!)

METHOD:

1. Preheat over to 200c and line a baking sheet with parchment paper.
2. Whisk together the eggs, cottage cheese and butter.
3. Separately, whisk the almond flour, garlic powder and salt before combining with the dry mixture from step 2. Then stir to combine.
4. Roll the resulting dough between two parchment paper sheets. The dough will be very wet, so you will need to peel the top parchment sheet off and bake it on the bottom sheet of parchment on a baking sheet.
5. Bake for 12-14 minutes or until it reaches your desired level of crispiness.
6. Add whatever sauces, toppings and cheese variants that you like and then bake for another 5-8 minutes or until the cheese has melted.

BREAKFAST

You're up, you're at it. Time to break your fast. Unless you're willing to put some graft in, or scour the planet for some of the few existing low-carb cereal brands out there, let's face it, cereals are more or less off the menu if you're going for a strict low carb diet. Whether you want fast and punchy or are up early enough to craft a mouth-watering masterpiece, in this section, we'll equip you with the skills so that you wake up excited to whip together a delicious and nutritious start to your day.

SALMON SPINACH SCRAMBLED

Easy, fast, packed with protein and delicious. What more could you want in a low carb day starter? This also works wonderfully with eggs benedict or baked eggs but if it's ease and speed you're after, we recommend scrambling. You can even swap your salmon out for bacon.

Nutrition:

Net carbs – 2g
Protein – 25g
Fat – 34g
Calories – 419

INGREDIENTS (FOR 2 SERVINGS):

- 1 tablespoon butter
- 2 tablespoon heavy whipping cream
- 30g baby spinach
- 60g smoked salmon or cooked bacon
- Salt and ground black pepper

METHOD:

1. Heat the butter in a frying pan. Add the baby spinach and fry until soft.
2. Add the whipping cream and let it bubble for a few moments until creamy.
3. Crack the eggs straight into the pan and stir so everything gets well incorporated.
4. Season with salt and pepper.
5. Keep stirring until everything is cooked how you like it.
6. Put the scrambled eggs on a plate and serve them together with smoked salmon or bacon.

SCALLION EGG MUFFINS

Explode your tastebuds into life this morning by piling the cheese, pesto and eggs onto some scallions. Delicious, certainly nutritious and not too much work.

Nutrition:

Net carbs – 2g
Protein – 26g
Fat – 26g
Calories – 353

Ingredients: (for 6 servings)

- 2 (30g) scallions, finely chopped
- 140g cooked bacon or salami, chopped
- 12 eggs
- 2 tablespoon red pesto or green pesto
- 170g grated cheddar cheese
- Salt and pepper

METHOD:

1. Preheat the oven to 175c.
2. You have three options here; place baking cups on a tray, grease a suitable tin with butter, or use a non-stick muffin tin (two muffins per serving).
3. Add scallions and the cooked bacon or salami to the bottom of the tin.
4. Whisk the eggs, salt, pesto and pepper together until combined.
5. Pour the resulting mixture on top of the scallions and meat.
6. Sprinkle some cheese on top.
7. Depending on the size of the tin, bake for 15-20 minutes.

VEGGIE SCRAMBLED EGGS

Want to learn how to make really bloomin' good scrambled eggs? Well, here you go.

Nutrition:

Net carbs – 4g
Protein – 32g
Fat – 34g
Calories – 455

INGREDIENTS (FOR 2 SERVINGS):

- 2 tablespoon butter
- 55g sliced mushrooms
- 6 eggs
- 55g red bell peppers, diced
- Salt and ground black pepper
- 120ml shredded parmesan cheese
- 1 (15g) chopped scallion

METHOD:

1. Heat the butter in a large pan before adding the mushrooms and red peppers. Season with salt and pepper and fry until soft.
2. Crack the eggs straight into the pan and stir right away so everything incorporates nicely.
3. Form large, soft curds by moving the spatula across the bottom and side of the pan. Cook until there is no more visible egg liquid but before they become dry.
4. Put it on a plate and top with shredded parmesan and scallions.

LEMON POPPY RICOTTA PANCAKES

Pancakes? PANCAKES?! Yep, pancakes. Pancakes that are so damn good for you and low in net carbs that you can munch on down whenever you like.

Nutrition:

Net carbs – 5.5g
Protein – 29.5g
Fat – 26g
Calories – 370

INGREDIENTS (FOR 4 SERVINGS):

- 2 large lemon, juiced and zested
- 6 large eggs
- ½ cup powdered erythritol
- ½ cup almond flour
- 2 scoop of egg white protein powder
- 300g whole milk ricotta
- 2 tablespoon heavy cream
- 2 tablespoon poppy seeds
- 20 to 24 drops liquid stevia
- 1½ teaspoons baking powder

METHOD:

1 Combine the ricotta, eggs, and liquid stevia in a blender with half the lemon juice and the lemon zest. Blend it well and truly before pouring into a bowl.
2 Create a dry mix by whisking together the poppy seeds, almond flour, baking powder and protein powder with a pinch of salt.
3 Heat a large non-stick pan over medium heat before spooning the batter into the pan, using about ¼ cup per pancake.
4 Fry the pancakes until bubbles form in the batter and then flip them, stylishly or not.
5 Let the pancakes cook until the bottom is browned then pop them on a plate.
6 Repeat with the remaining batter.
7 Whisk together the heavy cream, powdered erythritol, and reserved lemon juice and zest.
8 Serve the pancakes hot drizzled with the lemon glaze.

PEPPER JACK SAUSAGE EGG MUFFINS

Is there anything about that title that doesn't sound absolutely incredible?

Nutrition:

Net carbs – 3g
Protein – 26g
Fat – 37g
Calories – 455

INGREDIENTS (FOR 6 SERVINGS):

- 500g ground breakfast sausage
- 6 large eggs, whisked
- 1 cup diced yellow onion
- ½ teaspoon garlic powder
- Salt and pepper
- 1 cup shredded pepper jack cheese
- 4 tablespoons heavy cream

METHOD:

1. Preheat the oven to 175c and grease three ramekins with cooking spray.
2. Combine and stir the ground sausage, garlic powder, diced onion and sprinkle some salt and pepper in a mixing bowl.
3. Divide the sausage mixture evenly in the ramekins.
4. Pressing it into the bottom and sides, leaving an open space in the middle.
5. Separately whisk the eggs, heavy cream, salt and pepper together.
6. Divide the resulting mixture among the sausage cups and top with shredded cheese.
7. Bake for 25 to 30 minutes until the eggs are set and the cheese browned.

BACON BREAKFAST BOMBS

Bombs of bacon. They taste exactly how it sounds.

Nutrition:

Net carbs – 4.5g
Protein – 21g
Fat – 49g
Calories – 535

INGREDIENTS (FOR 4 SERVINGS OF 3 BOMBS):

- 8 slices thick-cut bacon
- 4 large eggs
- ½ cup cubed butter
- 4 tablespoons mayonnaise
- Salt and pepper

METHOD:

1 Cook the bacon in a large pan over medium-high heat until crisp.
2 Once cooked, allow the bacon to cool a little so that it's not too hot to handle. Then, chop it into small pieces and put it aside. Be sure to reserve the bacon grease as we don't want to miss out on extra tasty bits of fat now, do we?
3 Bring a pot of water to the boil. Add a pinch of salt.
4 Add the eggs and boil them for 10 minutes. Once cooked, transfer them into a separate pot of ice water.
5 Once the eggs have cooled, peel them and chop them tactlessly.
6 Mash the eggs with the butter then mix in the mayonnaise, salt, and pepper.
7 Stir in that excess bacon grease from earlier and cover the mixture, allowing it to chill for 30 minutes.
8 Divide the egg mixture in six portions and roll them into balls. Then roll in the crushed bacon that was set aside earlier.
9 Then you're ready to serve. Any leftovers, store in the fridge.

THE KETO FRY-UP

Fry-ups. What would life be without them? Don't worry, even though you've transitioned to keto, fry ups are going nowhere.

Nutrition:

Net carbs – 2g
Protein – 9g
Fat – 8g
Calories – 127

INGREDIENTS (FOR 4 SERVINGS):

- 4 eggs
- 4 large mushrooms
- 8 halved tomatoes
- 2 teaspoons of olive oil
- 200g spinach
- 1 thinly sliced garlic clove

(Be sure to add sausages, bacon and any other meat if you wish to make it a non-vegetarian breakfast!)

METHOD:

1 Heat the oven to 180c.
2 Using 4 ovenproof dishes, divide the mushrooms, tomatoes and garlic between them.
3 Season and drizzle oil over each of them before baking for 10 minutes.
4 While they bake, wilt the spinach by putting it in a colander and pour boiling water over it. Squeeze out the excess water and then add it to the dishes.
5 Create a space between the vegetables in each dish and then crack an egg into each gap.
6 Bake for a further 10 minutes or until the egg is cooked to your liking.

FAT-PACKED FRITTATA

Eat enough fat. It's very unlikely that you'll eat too much if your carb intake is low. This tasty bomb of a breakfast dish will give you a boost if you're not taking on enough fat.

Nutrition:

Net carbs – 4g
Protein – 25g
Fat – 34g
Calories – 433

INGREDIENTS (FOR 2 SERVINGS):

- 2 pork sausages
- 1 tablespoon of olive oil
- 3 large eggs
- 200g sliced mushrooms
- 100g asparagus
- 1 crushed garlic clove
- 1 tablespoon tarragon, chopped
- 1 tablespoon mustard
- 2 tablespoons full-fat soured cream
- (optional) Rocket salad mixture to serve

METHOD:

1. Preheat the grill to a high heat.
2. Meanwhile, in a medium-sized pan, heat the oil before adding mushrooms.
3. Crank the heat up and fry them for about 3 minutes.
4. Squeeze the meat out of the sausages and into little nuggets. Add them to the pan and fry them for another 5 minutes until they are golden brown.
5. Add the asparagus and the garlic before cooking for another minute or so.
6. Then, whip the soured cream, tarragon, mustard and the eggs into a jug and whisk them together.
7. Once whisked, season them how you like and pour the mixture into the pan.
8. Cook for about 3-4 minutes before grilling for a further 1-2 mins. The top should be just about set - there should be a slight wobble in the middle.
9. If you like, serve it with the salad leaves.

Cerealsly? You didn't think we'd *actually* let you go on living life without some kind of low-carb cereal option now, did you?

Nutrition:

Net carbs – 2g
Protein – 4g
Fat – 4g
Calories – 172

INGREDIENTS (FOR TEN 40G SERVINGS):

♦ 200g almond flour
♦ 1 egg
♦ 4 teaspoons ground cinnamon
♦ 100g erythritol
♦ 110g butter
♦ 1 teaspoon flax meal (or ½ teaspoon xanthan gum)
♦ ½ teaspoon baking soda
♦ ¼ teaspoon salt
♦ 2 tablespoons xylitol or Swerve

METHOD:

1   Whisk together cinnamon, almond flour, flax meal, salt and baking soda in a medium sized bowl until well combined. Set aside.

2   Mix the butter into a cream before adding the erythritol. Continue to whisk it until truly light and fluffy. Then incorporate the egg before adding half of the flour mixture from step 1. As it just begins to combine, add the remainder.

3   With it now resembling a dough, wrap in a film and refrigerate for between 1 hour and 3 days.

4   Then, whilst heating the oven to 180c, spread the dough between two pieces of parchment paper until it is thin. Cut straight lines length and crosswise into squares and then poke each piece with a fork.

5   Move the parchment paper to a tray and place in the freezer for 10 minutes before baking.

6   Bake for 8-12 minutes until it appears golden.

7   Smother with melted butter and sprinkle with cinnamon before allowing to cool for ten minutes before transferring to a cooling rack. The cereal should store in an airtight container for up to 5 days.

LUNCH

Sandwiches. Wraps. Soups. Salads. You know what lunch is. Find how to make your classic mid-day meals low carb, right here, right now.

BALT WRAPS

The BLT becomes the BALT. Pop some avocado in there and my oh my have you got a tasty sandwich. One of the best things to do for your gut is to replace the heavy, carb-filled bread that we typically wrap around our fillings with a crunchy, wholesome lettuce leaf. Get your seasonings and sauces right and you're onto a whole new world of wrapped up goodness!

Nutrition:

Net carbs – 4g
Protein – 31g
Fat – 53g
Calories – 631g

INGREDIENTS (FOR 2 SERVINGS):

- 170g sliced bacon
- 3 tablespoon mayonnaise
- 55g lettuce
- ½ avocado (100g)
- 1 sliced tomato (110g)
- Salt and pepper

METHOD:

1 On a medium heat fry the bacon in a large pan for about 5 minutes until it is crispy and then set it aside.
2 When cool enough to handle, cut each strip in half.
3 Squeeze a line of mayonnaise onto each of the lettuce leaves before adding a half-slice of tomato, 3 half-slices of bacon and a slice of avocado to each leaf.

SEAFOOD CHOWDER

You're on a boat, anchored in a calm sea while the sun sets. The sound of the captain pouring a glass of your favourite wine is followed by a burst of smell from the kitchen as the chef delivers you a wonderful dish. That's how good this tastes.

Nutrition:

Net carbs – 6g
Protein – 37g
Fat – 69g
Calories – 792

INGREDIENTS (FOR 3 SERVINGS):

- 3 tablespoon butter
- 1 ½ garlic cloves, minced
- 110g celery stalks
- 180ml clam juice
- 270ml heavy whipping cream
- 1 ½ teaspoon dried sage or dried thyme
- 2/5 lemon juice and zest
- 85g cream cheese
- 325g salmon, boneless fillets. You can use other fish but ensure it is boneless.
- 45g baby spinach
- 170g shrimp peeled and deveined
- Salt and ground black pepper
- 2/5 tablespoon red chilli peppers
- Fresh sage, optional for garnish

METHOD:

1   Melt butter in a large pot before adding garlic and celery.
2   Cook them for about 5 minutes with occasional stirring before adding clam juice, cream, cream cheese, sage, lemon juice and lemon zest. Let it simmer for 10 minutes without the lid.
3   Add the fish and shrimp before simmering until the fish is just about cooked. Then add the baby spinach and stir.
4   Season with salt and pepper before jazzing up the appearance with fresh red chilli and sage to garnish.

SESAME PORK LETTUCE WRAPS

I know using lettuce as a tortilla doesn't sound that exciting. But trust me, it provides a crunch and wholesomeness that bread just can't quite achieve. And when you're putting ingredients like these inside... Well. You're laughing.

Nutrition:

Net carbs – 7.5g
Protein – 49g
Fat – 29g
Calories – 500

INGREDIENTS (FOR 2 SERVINGS):

- 1 tablespoon olive oil
- ¼ cup diced green pepper
- 2 tablespoons diced celery
- 2 tablespoons soy sauce
- ¼ cup diced yellow onion
- 150g ground pork
- 1 tablespoon toasted sesame seed
- ¼ teaspoon onion powder
- ¼ teaspoon garlic powder
- 1 teaspoon sesame oil
- 4 leaves butter lettuce, separated

METHOD:

1 Heat the oil in a pan over medium heat.
2 Sauté the peppers, onions, and celery for about 5 minutes.
3 Mix in the pork and cook until it starts to turn brown.
4 Next, chuck in the onion powder and garlic powder then mix in the soy sauce and sesame oil.
5 Season with salt and pepper to taste before removing from the heat.
6 Put the lettuce leaves on a plate. Acting like a tortilla would, spoon the pork mixture into them evenly.
7 Sprinkle with sesame seeds to serve.

HAM AND CHEESE WAFFLES

Yep, Waffles! We typically think of waffles as an early morning, covered in syrup job. But no more. Savoury waffles are some of the best things I have ever tasted. I'd even recommend them with keto-fried chicken too, which you'll learn how to make later. But the simple beauty of Ham and Cheese is a real winner.

Nutrition:

Net carbs – 5g
Protein – 55g
Fat – 46.5g
Calories – 575

INGREDIENTS (FOR 4 SERVINGS):

- 4 scoops (40g) egg white protein powder
- 2 teaspoon baking powder
- 50g diced ham
- 8 large eggs, divided
- 2/3 cup melted butter
- 1 teaspoon salt
- ½ cup shredded cheddar cheese

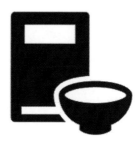

METHOD:

1 Separate the eggs into two halves.
2 Beat 4 of the egg yolks with the baking powder, protein powder, butter, and salt in a mixing bowl.
3 Mix in the chopped ham and pre-grated cheddar cheese.
4 Separately whisk the other egg whites in a bowl with a pinch of salt until stiff peaks form.
5 Mix the beaten egg whites into the egg yolk mixture in two batches. Meanwhile, preheat a waffle maker.
6 Grease the waffle maker then spoon ¼ cup of the batter into it and close it.
7 Cook for about 3 to 4 minutes until the waffle is golden brown.
8 Remove the waffle. Reheat the waffle iron and repeat with the remaining batter.
9 In the meantime, heat the oil in a pan and fry the eggs with salt and pepper.
10 Serve the waffles hot, topped with a fried egg.

CHEESEBURGER SALAD

Super easy. Super cheesy. Either make this into a tasty salad or put the graft in by making burger buns from the keto bread recipe. Up to you. Enjoy!

Nutrition:

Net carbs – 8g
Protein – 27.5g
Fat – 27.5g
Calories – 395

INGREDIENTS (FOR 2 SERVINGS):

- 175g ground beef
- 75g chopped romaine lettuce
- Salt and pepper
- ¼ cup shredded cheddar cheese
- 3 tablespoons mayonnaise
- 1 tablespoon diced pickle
- Pinch smoked paprika
- 1 teaspoon mustard
- 1/3 cup diced tomatoes
- ½ teaspoon ketchup

METHOD:

1. Cook the ground beef until brown over a high heat. Season with salt and pepper to taste.
2. Remove the pan from the heat and drain the fat.
3. Mix the mustard, paprika, pickles, ketchup, and mayonnaise in a blender and blend until smooth.
4. Syndicate the tomatoes, lettuce, and cheese in a bowl.
5. Toss in the ground beef and the dressing until evenly coated.

AVOCADO AND SALAMI SANDWICHES

Time to flip back to page one and make some keto-bread. If you haven't done it yet, you have to as it is life changing.

Nutrition:

Net carbs – 5g
Protein – 22.5g
Fat – 40.5g
Calories – 490

INGREDIENTS (FOR 4 SERVINGS):

- 4 keto bread buns
- 1 teaspoon butter
- 1 small avocado, sliced thin
- 1 medium tomato, sliced into 4 slices

- 25g fresh mozzarella, sliced thin
- 4 large eggs
- 50g sliced salami
- Salt and pepper

METHOD:

1 Follow our recipe in the "Keto Basics" section at the start of this book to prepare your bread.
2 Heat the butter in a large pan over medium heat.
3 Crack the eggs into the pan and season with salt and pepper.
4 Cook the eggs until done to the desired level then place one on each cloud bun.
5 Fill the buns with salami sliced tomato, avocado and, crucially, mozzarella.

SPRING SALAD WITH STEAK AND SWEET DRESSING

Raspberries, meet steak. Steak, meet raspberries. Believe it, it's delicious.

Nutrition:

Net carbs – 2.5g
Protein – 41g
Fat – 43.5g
Calories – 575

INGREDIENTS (FOR 2 SERVINGS):

- 175g beef flank steak
- 25g toasted pine nuts
- 2 tablespoons white wine vinegar
- 2 tablespoons olive oil
- 2 tablespoons fresh raspberries
- Liquid stevia
- 4 cups fresh spring greens
- 1 tablespoon butter
- 2 slices thick-cut bacon

METHOD:

1. Cook the bacon in a pan over medium-high heat until very crisp then chop fine.
2. Syndicate the liquid stevia, olive oil, white wine vinegar, and the almighty raspberries in a blender and blend until smooth.
3. Combine the crumbled bacon, spring greens and pine nuts in a large bowl.
4. Toss them all about, mixing them in nicely with the dressing before dividing between two plates.
5. Melt the butter in a heavy pan over medium-high heat then add the steak.
6. Season with salt and pepper then sear on one side, about 3 to 4 minutes.
7. Turn the steak over, cook it how you prefer and then allow it to rest for 5 minutes.
8. Cut the steak and divide it between the salads.

PEANUT BUTTER CHICKEN THIGHS

Peanut Butter. Chicken. Chicken and Peanut Butter. Together. I mean...
What more is there to say?

Nutrition:

Net carbs – 8g
Protein – 33g
Fat – 43g
Calories – 572

INGREDIENTS (FOR 4 SERVINGS):

- 2 tablespoons of vegetable oil
- 8 skinless boneless chicken thighs
- 1 finely chopped onion
- 3 crushed garlic cloves
- 2 finely sliced red chillies
- 2 teaspoons of grated fresh ginger
- 2 tablespoons of garam masala
- 100g peanut butter
- 400ml coconut milk
- 400g can chopped tomatoes
- Roughly chopped coriander
- Picked leaves of coriander
- Roasted peanuts
- (option of adding cauliflower rice – ensure to add to the carb count though)

METHOD:

1 In a frying pan over a medium heat, heat 1 tablespoon of the oil.
2 Cut the chicken into chunks and brown it in batches. Set aside once golden.
3 Fry the onion until it has softened - for about 8 minutes.
4 Add the ginger, chilli, garlic and another tablespoon of oil and then fry for 1 minute.
5 Add the garam masala and keep frying for a further minute.
6 Mix in the tomatoes, coconut milk and peanut butter before bringing it all to a simmer.
7 Pop the chicken back in the pan and sling in the chopped coriander.
8 Cook until the sauce has thickened and the chicken is cooked through (about another 30 minutes).
9 During this time, you can prepare your cauliflower rice if you wish.
10 Serve with the roasted peanuts and coriander.

PROTEIN-PACKED PESTO SALAD

Chicken, broccoli, avocado and beetroot combine with pesto to make this absolute king of a salad. Enjoy feeling great.

Nutrition:

Net carbs – 2g
Protein – 29g
Fat – 18g
Calories – 320

INGREDIENTS (FOR 4 SERVINGS):

- 250g thin-stemmed broccoli
- 3 skinless chicken breasts
- 1 sliced red onion
- 2 teaspoons rapeseed oil

- 2 peeled raw beetroots
- 1 teaspoon nigella seeds
- 100g watercress

For the pesto:
- 1 avocado
- 1/2 crushed garlic cloves
- 25g crumbled walnut halves
- Small packet of basil
- 1 lemon juiced and zested
- 1 tablespoon of rapeseed oil

METHOD:

1 Boil a large pan of water and then add the broccoli for about 2 minutes and then drain and refresh.

2 Throw the broccoli in a heated pan along with ½ teaspoon of the oil and sizzle for 2-3 minutes.

3 Set it aside to cool and slap the remaining oil and seasonings onto the chicken before cooking for about 3-4 minutes until it's cooked through. Leave it to cool and then cut it into chunks.

4 To make the pesto, pick the basil leaves, putting some into a blender and setting some of them aside for later. Scoop the core of the avocado into the blender too, along with the walnuts, garlic, a tablespoon of lemon, some seasoning and 2-3 tablespoons of cold water. Blend it until smooth and transfer to a small serving dish.

5 Pour lemon juice over the sliced onions and allow them time to soak in.

6 Toss the broccoli, watercress, and the lemon/ onion combination together on a large plate and then top with the beetroot and chicken without mixing it in.

7 Sprinkle the remaining basil leaves, lemon zest, nigella seeds and serve with the pesto.

BOUYIOURDI

Boy are you ready for Bouyriourdi! Nearly works. Time to venture into Greek cuisine with this superb baked feta meze.

Nutrition:

Net carbs – 3g
Protein – 8g
Fat – 21g
Calories – 243

INGREDIENTS (FOR 4 SERVINGS):

- 200g feta
- 3 large tomatoes
- 1 sliced large green chilli or pepper
- 1 crushed garlic clove
- 4 tablespoons olive oil
- 1 teaspoon chopped oregano leaves

METHOD:

1. Cut 2 central slices of tomato and set aside.
2. Spoon out the seeds from the rest of the tomato and then grate the flesh. Get rid of the skin. Follow this process with the rest of the tomatoes and then mix the grated skin with the garlic before seasoning and scooping into a baking dish.
3. Heat the oven the 200c.
4. Pop the block of feta in with the tomato/garlic mixture and add the chilli, sliced tomatoes, salt, olive oil and oregano.
5. Cover and bake for 15 minutes before uncovering and baking for a further 15.
6. Serve warm, with the option of adding keto bread for dipping and dunking.

DINNER

If we're lucky, we may occasionally cook a lover some breakfast. You may even have some friends round for a spot of lunch. But as we all know, the pressure of wanting to perform in the kitchen tends to focus around probably the most exciting meal of all. Dinner time. As a dedicated keto person – you will likely experience doubters and naysayers giving you jip for your disciplined lifestyle. Well, in this section, you're going to be equipped with the arsenal to fend off any keto-critics, knowing whole heartedly that you can whip up dishes left right and centre if ever you needed to prove the exciting and flavourful ways of keto-life.

KETO SPAGHETTI MEATBALLS

Yep. Meatballs. As mentioned below, you can even add bean pasta to this dish to get the classic spaghetti meatballs combination that is quite rightly something you don't want to give up.

Nutrition:

Net carbs – 5g
Protein – 39g
Fat – 49g
Calories – 628

INGREDIENTS (FOR 4 SERVINGS):
- 450g ground beef or turkey
- 60g shredded Parmesan cheese
- 1 egg
- 1teaspoon salt
- ½ tablespoon dried basil
- ½ teaspoon onion powder
- 1 teaspoon garlic powder
- ½ teaspoon ground black pepper
- 3 tablespoon olive oil
- 425g tinned whole tomatoes
- 2 tablespoon fresh parsley, finely chopped
- 200g fresh spinach
- 55g butter
- 140g fresh mozzarella cheese
- Salt and pepper
- (option to add the bean pasta we mentioned earlier!)

METHOD:

1 Put the ground beef, egg, salt, spices and the parmesan cheese into a bowl and blend or whish thoroughly. Keep your hands wet and from the resulting mixture, form meatballs about 30g each.

2 Heat the olive oil in a large pan and move the meatballs around until they're golden brown on all sides.

3 Lower the heat and add the canned tomatoes before letting it simmer for 15 minutes with the occasional stir.

4 Season with salt and pepper. Add parsley and continue stirring.

5 Melt butter in a separate frying pan and fry the spinach, stirring continuously.

6 Add salt and pepper to taste before combining the spinach with the meatballs.

7 Tear mozzarella into bite sized pieces and serve it on top.

CHICKEN BURGER WITH JALAPENO AIOLI

Again, the power of the lettuce leaf comes to the fore as burgers remain on the menu with a delicious alternative to the bun. Of course, if you're craving the wholesome texture of a burger bun, whip to our bread replacement page and learn how to cook your very own keto bread!

Nutrition:

Net carbs – 3g
Protein – 31g
Fat – 35g
Calories – 460

INGREDIENTS (FOR 4 SERVINGS):

- 450g chicken breasts
- 2 tablespoon butter
- Salt and ground black pepper
- 8 butterhead lettuce leaves

- 4 slices cheddar cheese
- ½ sliced onion (55g)
- 1 sliced tomato (110g)

For the aioli:

- 120ml mayonnaise
- 2tablespoon pickled jalapenos, minced
- 1 garlic clove, minced
- Salt and ground black pepper to taste

METHOD:

1. Trim and wash the lettuce leaves. Slice the tomato and the onion.
2. Mix the ingredients for the aioli together in a small bowl and set it aside.
3. Cut the chicken breasts into halves or thirds depending on their size. Add plenty of salt and pepper to season.
4. Sizzle the butter in a large pan on a medium heat and then add the sliced chicken. Fry on both sides until cooked throughout.
5. Lower the heat, place the cheese on top of the chicken and continue frying until the cheese begins to melt.
6. Add a lettuce leaf to each plate before placing the chicken on top, followed by a dollop of the jalapeno aioli, some tomato and some onion. Pop another salad leaf on there to finish it off.

TUNA BURGERS

Tuna, egg, crunchy greens and veg – this burger is crammed with protein and will keep you satisfied for quite some time. Straight forward preparation and a delicious end product. Enjoy.

Nutrition:

Net carbs – 8g
Protein – 39g
Fat – 58g
Calories – 722

INGREDIENTS (FOR 2 SERVINGS):

- 280g drained tinned tuna
- 90ml mayonnaise
- 1 large egg
- 1 tablespoon garlic powder
- 1 tablespoon onion powder
- ¼ teaspoon salt
- ¼ teaspoon ground black pepper
- 1 ½ tablespoon olive oil
- 1 sliced tomato (100g)
- 45g leafy greens or lettuce
- 2 tablespoon mayonnaise

METHOD:

1 Combine all the ingredients together except the oil in a medium-sized bowl.
2 Shape the mixture into small burgers about 5cm wide and 1cm thick.
3 Pan-fry the burgers one at a time. Add plenty of oil so that it coats the base of a large frying pan. When the oil is hot, place the tuna patties in the pan.
4 Cook for 3-4 minutes until golden-brown and crispy. Occasionally press the sides lightly with a spatula.
5 To serve, add a few lettuce leaves to each plate and top each leaf with a tuna burger, tomato slice and a dollop of mayonnaise.
6 Salt and pepper to taste.

ASIAN STYLE CHICKEN STIR-FRY WITH BROCCOLI

Asian cuisine is certainly not off the menu, and we're going to give you an unbelievable stir fry to keep you in check with it.

Nutrition:

Net carbs – 5g
Protein – 43g
Fat – 46g
Calories – 613

INGREDIENTS (2 SERVINGS):

- 400g boneless chicken thighs
- 140g broccoli, trimmed into small pieces
- ½ teaspoon ground black pepper
- ½ teaspoon garlic powder
- 1 tablespoon tamari soy sauce
- 1 tablespoon olive oil or coconut oil

For the mayonnaise:

- 90 ml mayonnaise
- 1 tablespoon hot sauce
- ½ teaspoon garlic powder

METHOD:

1   For the mayonnaise, combine all the ingredients in a small bowl and stir before setting aside.
2   Heat the oil in a wok or large pan.
3   Add the chicken, garlic powder and pepper. Stir-fry for a few minutes, until the chicken turns golden brown.
4   Add the broccoli and tamari soy sauce. Move it all around until the broccoli becomes crisp as you stir.
5   Spoon into individual bowls and serve with the spicy mayonnaise on the side.

CRACK CHICKEN IN THE KETO KITCHEN

Don't be forgetting to cook crack chicken in your keto kitchen. Too good to resist. Just like those rhymes... Cream cheese. Cheddar cheese. Bacon. The beauty of not having to hold back your fat intake comes to the fore in this scrumptious recipe.

Nutrition:

Net carbs – 4g
Protein – 50g
Fat – 35g
Calories – 537

INGREDIENTS (FOR 4 SERVINGS):

- 600g chicken breasts
- 1 tablespoon ranch seasoning
- 1 1/3 tablespoon fresh chives, chopped
- 2/3 teaspoon salt
- 95g diced bacon
- 75g cheddar cheese
- 190g cream cheese
- 60g baby spinach
- 1/6 teaspoon ground black pepper

METHOD:

1. Combine the ranch seasoning, salt and cream cheese in a bowl before placing the chicken in the bottom of the slow cooker.
2. Spread out the cream cheese mix on top of the chicken.
3. Once covered with the lid, either select the low setting of 5 hours or the high of 3 hours.
4. Fry the bacon in a frying pan until crispy before setting aside.
5. Shred the chicken and then mix everything together. Dust some cheese and bacon on top before covering with the lid until the cheese melts.
6. Sprinkle chives and black pepper before serving with baby spinach.

SAUSAGE AND CABBAGE SKILLET

It takes pan to cook a pan. It's actually pretty simple but I just like that sentence. Enjoy.

Nutrition:

Net carbs – 10g
Protein – 22g
Fat – 24.5g
Calories – 350

INGREDIENTS (FOR 4 SERVINGS):

- 6 large Italian sausage links
- ¼ cup mayonnaise
- 2 tablespoons butter
- ¼ cup sour cream
- Salt and pepper
- ½ head green cabbage, sliced

METHOD:

1. Cook the sausage in a pan over medium-high heat until evenly browned then slice them.
2. Reheat the pan over medium-high heat then add the butter.
3. Mix in the cabbage and cook for about 3 to 4 minutes until it is wilted.
4. Stir the sliced sausage into the cabbage then chuck in the sour cream and mayonnaise and mix it all.
5. For seasoning, sprinkle with salt and pepper then keep everything simmering on a low temperature for 10 minutes.

BEEF BILTONG CHILLI-CON-CARNE

Chilli con carne with a twist. Sling this in a lettuce tortilla, or chuck it over cauliflower rice and you've brought chilli con carne into your keto life.

Nutrition:

Net carbs – 10g
Protein – 45g
Fat – 27g
Calories – 502

INGREDIENTS (FOR 4 SERVINGS):

- 100g biltong
- 1 sliced, large onion
- 2 tablespoons of sunflower oil
- 400g beef mince
- 1 tablespoon cumin seeds
- 1 tablespoon ground coriander
- 4 tablespoons of chipotle paste
- 600ml beef stock
- 400g can of kidney beans. Drain but don't rinse.
- 2 juiced limes. Use the zest of 1.
- Cayenne pepper
- 100g grated smoked cheddar
- Sliced jalapeno chillies
- Coriander leaves
- Optional cauliflower rice or lettuce tortillas (add to carb count!)

METHOD:

1. Blend the biltong to as fine a powder as you can and then set it aside in a bowl.
2. Spread the onion in a dry pan and cook on a low heat until dark and soft (for about 30 minutes).
3. During this time, heat oil in a pan and pop in the mince.
4. While cooking on a low heat for about 30 minutes, its own fat will help it to cook. If the pan is too dry however, pop in a bit more oil.
5. When the mince is nearing completion, stir it until brown crispy bits emerge.
6. Stir in the chipotle paste, coriander, beef stock and the cumin and then simmer for another 10 minutes.
7. Blend the caramelized onions until smooth and then, along with the biltong and the beans, add the resulting puree into the chilli.
8. Keep it on a low heat for a bit longer as you season with cayenne and lime juice.
9. Spoon the chilli into a bowl and dust the cheese, jalapenos and remaining biltong over the top. Garnish with lime zest and coriander leaves.

CAULIFLOWER STEAKS

This is one for the vegans. Our hats are well and truly tipped to those of you keto-vegans. Being a keto-vegan is a challenge, but certainly doable. Even if you're not vegan, get this tasty, nutritious recipe locked into your repertoire.

Nutrition:

Net carbs – 7g
Protein – 9g
Fat – 21g
Calories – 277

INGREDIENTS (FOR 2 SERVINGS):

- 1 roasted red pepper
- 1 cauliflower floret
- 2 tablespoons olive oil
- Small handful of parsley
- 4 pitted black olives
- ½ teaspoon smoked paprika
- 1 teaspoon of capers
- 2 tablespoons of flaked almonds
- ½ tablespoon of red wine vinegar

METHOD:

1. Line a baking tray with baking parchment and preheat the oven to 200c.
2. Cut the cauliflower floret into 2 1-inch-thick steaks. Our advice is to use the middle part because it is larger and save the rest of the floret for another time (such as cauliflower rice).
3. Smother the steaks with ½ a tablespoon of oil and paprika and then season how you like.
4. Pop them on a tray and cook them for 15-20 minutes.
5. Meanwhile, prepare the salsa.
6. Cut the parsley, capers, olives and peppers and then put them in a bowl. Mix with the remaining 1½ tablespoons of oil and the vinegar before seasoning.
7. Once the steaks are cooked through, pop the salsa and flaked almonds on top and serve.

MUSSELS CURRY

Nutrition:

Net carbs – 8g
Protein – 14g
Fat – 23g
Calories – 292

INGREDIENTS (FOR 4 SERVINGS):

- 1kg of mussels
- 1 teaspoon of black mustard seed
- 2 teaspoons of ground coriander
- 2 chopped green chillies
- 1 chopped onion
- Salt and pepper
- ½ teaspoon ground turmeric
- 4 crushed garlic cloves
- Sunflower oil
- Grated ginger
- 400ml coconut milk
- Coriander sprigs and lime wedges (for garnish)
- Option to add cauliflower rice (add to the carb count!)

METHOD:

1 Pick off the beards of the mussels and then wash them in cold water. Repeatedly refresh the water until it is clear, throwing away and muscles that are broken.
2 Using a casserole, heat the oil.
3 Fry the onion until it starts to brown before adding the garlic, spices, chillies, salt, pepper and ginger.
4 Cook everything together until it is fragrant – about 2-3 minutes.
5 Send in the coconut milk and then once it is boiling, simmer for a few minutes.
6 Next, in go the mussels before you cover it and crank the heat up to the maximum, boiling for 3-4 minutes until the mussels open.
7 Evenly distribute the coriander sprigs and serve with lime wedges on the side and maybe even cauliflower rice.

Matthew Josh

KETO SHEPHERD'S PIE

Shepherd's pie is great. There's no denying that. But something even better comes out of this recipe. Something that can transform your life in ketosis. Cauliflower mash. Easy. Simple. Here we go.

Nutrition:

Net carbs – 12g
Protein – 25g
Fat – 42g
Calories – 545

INGREDIENTS (FOR 4 SERVINGS):

For the cauliflower mash:
- 1 large cauliflower head
- 2 tablespoons of butter
- 2 tablespoons of cream cheese
- 4 cloves of garlic
- ¾ teaspoon of salt

For the pie:
- 2 tablespoons of olive oil
- 1 small, diced onion
- 64g diced carrots
- 1 diced green bell pepper
- 450g Ground lamb (or beef for cottage pie!)
- Salt and pepper
- 250ml Beef bone broth
- 1 tablespoon of coconut aminos
- 2 tablespoons of tomato paste

METHOD:

1. Starting with the cauliflower mash, cut the cauliflower into florets and put them in a large bowl with about 120ml water and then cover with a plastic wrap.

2. Microwave for 10-15 minutes until it's mushy and soft, and then drain it before blending with all the ingredients for about 2 minutes until it becomes smooth like a puree.

3. Add salt and pepper to taste before setting aside.

4. Heat the oven to 200c.

5. Heat the oil in a large pan over medium heat, and then sauté the peppers, carrots and onions until browned (about 6-10 minutes).

6. Move the vegetables to the side of the pan and add in the ground lamb. Add salt and pepper to season and cook until the meat is brown.

7. Mix in the tomato paste, coconut aminos, the broth, and any additional seasonings desired. Once boiling, simmer uncovered until most of the liquid evaporates and the sauce thickens. This should take about 5 minutes, and then remove it from the heat.

8. Evenly spread the mashed cauliflower on top with a rubber spatula and then bake for 10-15 minutes.

21-DAY KETO DIET PLAN

There we have it. You're equipped with recipes to not only keep you thin, fit and firing, but to whip up a storm in the kitchen that even your non-keto friends will be pleasantly shocked by. Now it's time to get you rolling with your very own keto diet plan. This 21-day plan will either kick-start your keto life with a bang, or give you that extra bit of structure that you're after to keep you on track.

We've put together a balanced diet plan that will provide you with all the nutrition you need to keep lean while performing mentally, and all those other benefits we spoke of earlier. Each day you'll use two of the recipes already detailed within the book plus one new recipe per day to keep things fresh and exciting.

So, without further ado, let's get cooking. Welcome to the keto life.

DAY 1 NET CARBS – 13G

Day 1 kicks you off with a brilliant bundle of healthy dishes. Starting the day with the scrambled eggs and salmon combination, ending it with the phenomenal keto spaghetti meatballs, with a fresh lunch wedged in the middle there. This spice pumpkin soup is to die for. It might not be a bad idea to prepare some of the keto bread that we recommended too because we ensure you, you'll want to wipe up every last drop of this sumptuous soup.

Even if you are aiming for the strictest of the keto diets (below 25g net carbs per day) then day 1's diet plan still allows you the room to squeeze in some sneaky low-carb snacks if you'd like!

Breakfast: Salmon Spinach Scrambled (See page 28)

Lunch: Spiced Pumpkin Soup

Dinner: Keto Spaghetti Meatballs (See page 53)

SPICED PUMPKIN SOUP

Nutrition:

Net Carbs – 6g
Protein – 10g
Fat – 20g
Calories – 250

INGREDIENTS (FOR 6 SERVINGS):

- 4 tablespoons unsalted butter
- 1 cup pumpkin puree
- 2 small, chopped yellow onion
- 4 cloves garlic, minced
- 2 teaspoon minced ginger
- 2 cup chicken broth
- 1 teaspoon ground cinnamon
- ½ teaspoon ground nutmeg
- Salt and pepper to taste
- 6 slices thick-cut bacon
- ½ cup heavy cream

METHOD:

1   Put the butter in a large pan over medium heat until it melts.
2   Add the garlic, onions and ginger. Cook for 3 to 4 minutes until the onions are transparent.
3   Mix in the spices and cook for 1 minute until a nice fragrance emerges. Add salt and pepper.
4   Pop in the chicken broth and the pumpkin puree and then bring to a boil.
5   Reduce the heat and simmer for 20 minutes before removing from the heat.
6   Using a blender, make the soup into a puree before returning it to heat and simmer for 20 minutes.
7   Cook the bacon in a separate pan until crisp. Then remove it onto paper towels and allow it to drain.
8   Along with the heavy cream, add the bacon fat to the soup and then crumble the bacon over the top to serve.

DAY 2 NET CARBS – 25G

Okay so today we're giving you a breakfast recipe that has a slightly higher net carb intake. With lunch and dinner low in net carbs though, it balances out and keeps you below the 25g daily net carb marker. Cereal lovers, this one's for you.

Breakfast: Sweet Blueberry Coconut Porridge

Lunch: BALT Wraps (See page 39)

Dinner: Asian Style Chicken Stir-fry with Broccoli (See page 58)

SWEET BLUEBERRY COCONUT PORRIDGE

Nutrition:

Net carbs – 15g
Protein – 10g
Fat – 22g
Calories – 390

INGREDIENTS (FOR 2 SERVINGS):

- ♦ ¼ cup coconut flour
- ♦ ¼ cup ground flaxseed
- ♦ ¼ teaspoon ground nutmeg
- ♦ Pinch of salt
- ♦ 1 cup unsweetened almond milk
- ♦ ¼ cup canned coconut milk
- ♦ 60 grams fresh blueberries
- ♦ ¼ cup shaved coconut
- ♦ 1 teaspoon ground cinnamon

METHOD:

1 Heat the almond milk and coconut milk in a saucepan over low heat until it is warm.
2 Whisk the flaxseed, cinnamon, nutmeg, coconut flour, and salt together.
3 Crank up the heat and cook everything together until the mixture bubbles.
4 Add in the sweetener and vanilla extract then stir while cooking until it thickens to your desired level.
5 Divide into two bowls before topping with blueberries and shaved coconut for a delicious bowl of porridge.

DAY 3 NET CARBS – 17G

An absolute winner of a breakfast dish, followed by a simple salad for lunch and Stir fry for dinner.

Breakfast: Chorizo Breakfast Bake

Lunch: Avocado and Salami Sandwiches (See page 45)

Dinner: Cauliflower Steaks (See page 63)

CHORIZO BREAKFAST BAKE

Nutrition:

Net carbs – 4.5
Protein – 25g
Fat – 36g
Calories – 450

INGREDIENTS (FOR 4 SERVINGS):

- 2 tablespoon olive oil
- 1 cup diced red pepper
- 1 cup diced yellow onion
- 200g chorizo sausage
- 4 large eggs
- Salt and pepper
- 4 slices thick-cut bacon, cooked

METHOD:

1. Preheat the oven to 175c and grease two ramekins.
2. Over a medium heat, heat the oil in a pan.
3. Throw in the peppers and onions and sizzle them for 4 to 5 minutes until they turn brown.
4. Split the vegetable mixture into the two ramekins.
5. Cut the chorizo and do the same between the ramekins.
6. Crack an egg into each ramekin.
7. Season with salt and pepper.
8. Bake for 10 to 12 minutes or until the egg is set to how you like it.
9. Put the crumbled bacon on top and serve.

DAY 4 NET CARBS – 17G

Bish, bash, bosh. Beef curry. Enjoy your day.
Breakfast: Veggie Scrambled Eggs (See page 30)
Lunch: Seafood Chowder (See page 40)
Dinner: Beef Curry

BEEF CURRY

Nutrition:

Net carbs – 9g
Protein – 50g
Fat – 34g
Calories – 550

INGREDIENTS (FOR 6 SERVINGS):

- 900g beef chuck, chopped
- 2½ cups canned coconut milk
- 2 medium onion, chopped
- 2 tablespoon garlic, minced
- 2 tablespoon grated ginger
- 4 tablespoons curry powder
- 2 teaspoon salt
- 1 cup fresh chopped coriander

You can always add cauliflower rice for the extra curry experience. Just be sure to acknowledge the extra net carbs.

METHOD:

1   Mix the garlic, onion and ginger in a blender until it comes to a paste.
2   Transfer the contents into a pan. Cook for 3 minutes on a medium heat.
3   Stir in the coconut milk then simmer gently for 10 minutes.
4   Then add the chopped beef as well as the curry powder and salt.
5   Stir well. Then pop the cover on and simmer for 20 minutes.
6   Once that's finished, simmer for another 20 minutes with the lid removed until the beef is cooked through.
7   Play with the seasonings, adjusting it to how you like it. Garnish with fresh chopped coriander.

DAY 5 NET CARBS – 16G

A scrumptious steak salad will drive home the protein. On about day 5 you should be starting to notice one or two changes in the body. Stay observant and keep asking your body what it needs.

Breakfast: Scallion Egg Muffins (See page 29)

Lunch: Garlic Steak Salad

Dinner: Sausage and Cabbage Skillet (See page 60)

GARLIC STEAK SALAD

Nutrition:

Net carbs – 6g
Protein – 52g
Fat – 48g
Calories – 681

Usually, the word salad sounds kind of bland. Not this one.

INGREDIENTS (FOR 2 SERVINGS):

- 450g flank, ribeye or sirloin steak cut into 2.5cm pieces
- 1 tablespoon ghee or butter
- 1 ½ finely chopped garlic cloves
- Salt and ground black pepper

- 110g leafy greens
- 110g cherry tomatoes
- ½ avocado
- 85g cucumber

For the dressing:
- 40ml mayonnaise
- 1 tablespoon water
- ¼ tablespoon dried tarragon
- ¼ tablespoon Dijon mustard
- ½ pressed garlic clove

METHOD:

1 Whip together the dressing ingredients and pop them in the fridge and prep the salad as you please.
2 Heat a large frying pan before adding the ghee or butter.
3 When melted, add the meat and splash on a wealthy amount of salt and pepper for seasoning.
4 When the meat starts to get some colour, add the garlic and mix it all around. Without overcooking, fry just until the meat is browned on all sides.
5 Sling the steak bites, garlic and meat juices from the pan into the salad before drizzling the dressing on top or serve it on the side.

DAY 6 NET CARBS – 16.5G

If I were you, I'd be very excited for dinner today. These stuffed aubergine boats are a dream.

Breakfast: Fat-packed Frittata (See page 35)

Lunch: Sesame Pork Lettuce Wraps (See page 41)

Dinner: Stuffed Aubergine Boats

STUFFED AUBERGINE BOATS

Nutrition:

Net carbs – 5g
Protein – 31g
Fat – 48g
Calories – 578

INGREDIENTS (3 SERVINGS):

- 325g ground beef or turkey
- 1 ½ tablespoon olive oil or butter
- ¾ teaspoon salt
- 1 ½ tablespoon Tex-Mex seasoning
- ¾ teaspoon salt
- 6g finely chopped fresh cilantro
- 1 ½ aubergine
- ¾ tablespoon olive oil
- 85g Shredded pepper Jack cheese
- 150g lettuce
- 3 tablespoon olive oil
- 2/5 tablespoon red wine vinegar or white vinegar
- Salt and pepper

METHOD:

1 Preheat the oven to 200c.
2 Cut the aubergines in half, remove the seeds and sprinkle with salt.
3 Allow the aubergine to sit for ten minutes. While they sit, brown the ground meat in an oiled pan. Add salt and the Tex-Mex seasoning and allow it to cook until most of the liquid has evaporated.
4 Dab the drops of excess liquid with paper towels. Place the aubergine halves in a greased baking dish.
5 Mix a third of the cheese into the ground beef and add the chopped cilantro.
6 Divide the resulting mixture evenly among the aubergine boats before sprinkling the remaining cheese on top.
7 Bake in the oven for about 20 minutes, or until the cheese begins to brown. Take the aubergine out and let it cool for five minutes.
8 Meanwhile, mix oil, vinegar, salt and pepper into a vinaigrette. Prep the salad and serve it alongside the aubergine boats.

DAY 7 NET CARBS – 20.5G

Start your day with a bang with this incredible low-carb vanilla smoothie.

Breakfast: Vanilla Protein Smoothie

Lunch: Ham and Cheese Waffles (See page 42)

Dinner: Mussels Curry (See page 64)

VANILLA PROTEIN SMOOTHIE

Nutrition:

Net carbs – 7.5g
Protein – 25g
Fat – 46g
Calories – 540

INGREDIENTS (2 SMOOTHIES):

- 2 scoops (about 40g) vanilla egg white protein powder
- 1 cup heavy cream
- ½ cup whipped cream
- ½ cup vanilla almond milk
- 8 ice cubes
- 2 tablespoon powdered erythritol
- 2 tablespoon coconut oil
- 1 teaspoon vanilla extract

METHOD:

1. Excluding the whipped cream, combine all of the ingredients in a blender and blend on high speed until smooth (about 30-60 seconds).
2. Transfer into a glass and top with whipped cream. Boom. Done.

DAY 8 NET CARBS – 25G

Now we're going to shuffle things round here to make space for this killer quiche. It's about as high in net carbs as you'd ever want to go, but work it in with some super low carb meals and you're good. No one wants to live a life without quiche, right?

Breakfast: Scallion Egg Muffins (See page 29)

Lunch: Mozzarella Veggie Quiche

Dinner: Chicken Burger with Jalapeno Aioli (See page 55)

MOZZARELLA VEGGIE QUICHE

Nutrition:

Net carbs – 17g
Protein – 38g
Fat – 40g
Calories – 590

INGREDIENTS (FOR 1 WHOLE QUICHE):
- ♦ 1 tablespoon grated parmesan cheese
- ♦ 2 slices thick-cut bacon
- ♦ 1 tablespoon heavy cream
- ♦ 1 teaspoon chopped chives
- ♦ ¼ cup spinach
- ♦ ¼ cup diced courgette
- ♦ ¼ cup shredded mozzarella cheese
- ♦ 2 large eggs, divided
- ♦ 4 cherry tomatoes, halved
- ♦ 6 tablespoons almond flour

METHOD:

1   Mix together the grated parmesan, almond flour, one egg and a pinch of salt until it becomes a soft dough.

2   As evenly as possible, press the dough into the bottom of a small, quiche shaped pan.

3   Make shallow cuts in the bottom and sides of the dough before baking for 7 minutes at 160c.

4   Then let it cool.

5   Cook the bacon in a pan until browned and then crumble and spread it into the quiche pan.

6   Throw in the spinach, courgette, cheese, and tomatoes.

7   With all the remaining egg, whisk it together with the heavy cream, chives, salt and pepper then pour into the quiche. Bake for about 25 minutes, ensuring that the egg is set. Serve while hot.

DAY 9 NET CARBS – 14.5G

Pancakes for breakfast. Waffles for lunch. You're welcome.

Breakfast: Lemon Poppy Ricotta Pancakes (See page 31)

Lunch: Ham and Cheese Waffles (See page 42)

Dinner: Avocado Lime Salmon

AVOCADO LIME SALMON

Nutrition:

Net carbs – 4g
Protein – 36g
Fat – 44g
Calories – 570

INGREDIENTS (FOR 2 SERVINGS):

- 100g chopped cauliflower rice
- 1 large avocado
- 1 tablespoon fresh lime juice
- 150g boneless salmon fillets
- 2 tablespoons diced red onion
- 2 tablespoons olive oil
- Salt and pepper

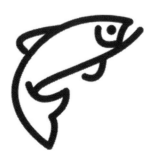

METHOD:

1. Either use our cauliflower rice recipe from earlier, or simply blend, chop or grate the cauliflower into rice-like grains.
2. Grease a pan and heat over medium heat.
3. Add the cauliflower rice and cook, covered, for 8 minutes until tender. Set aside.
4. Combine the avocado, lime juice and red onion in a food processor and blend until smooth.
5. In a large pan over medium heat, heat the oil.
6. Season the salmon with salt and pepper then add to the pan skin-side down.
7. Cook for 4 to 5 minutes on each side until baked.
8. Serve the salmon over the cauliflower rice and then top with the avocado cream.

DAY 10 NET CARBS – 17G

Happy omelette day.

Breakfast: Creamy Cheese Omelette

Lunch: Cheeseburger Salad (See page 44)

Dinner: Crack Chicken in the Keto Kitchen (See page 59)

CREAMY CHEESE OMELETTE

Nutrition:

Net carbs – 5g
Protein – 39g
Fat – 38g
Calories – 610

INGREDIENTS (FOR 1 SERVING):

- 2 eggs
- 2 tablespoon heavy whipping cream, salt and ground black pepper
- ½ tablespoon butter or coconut oil
- 85g shredded cheddar cheese

Filling ingredients:

- 2 sliced mushrooms
- 2 sliced cherry tomatoes
- 15g baby spinach
- 1 teaspoon dried oregano
- 2 tablespoon cream cheese
- 28g deli turkey

METHOD:

1 Beat the eggs and cream together in a bowl before seasoning with salt and pepper.

2 Melt the butter in a frying pan before spreading the cheese in an even layer in the pan so that it covers the entire bottom.

3 Pour the egg mixture over the cheese and lower the heat and then cook for a few minutes without stirring.

4 Fill one of the halves with mushrooms, tomatoes baby spice, cream cheese, turkey and oregano before frying for a few more minutes.

5 You can allow the mixture to be a bit loose on top – but not too loose! Once it has set, turn the empty half over the topping side, forming a crescent. Fry for a few more minutes and dig in!

DAY II NET CARBS – 17.5G

Prepare yourself for the snazziest salad you've had in quite some time. Meanwhile, Avo-Tzatziki will transform your life.

Breakfast: Salmon Spinach Scrambled (See page 28)

Lunch: Gyro Salad with Avo-Tzatziki

Dinner: Tuna Burgers (See page 57)

GYRO SALAD WITH AVO-TZATZIKI

Nutrition:

Net carbs – 7.5g
Protein – 45g
Fat – 29g
Calories – 495

INGREDIENTS (FOR 3 SERVINGS):

- ♦ 450g ground lamb meat
- ♦ 1 tablespoon olive oil
- ♦ ½ teaspoon dried oregano
- ♦ ½ teaspoon dried thyme
- ♦ ½ medium sized onion, diced
- ♦ ¼ cup chicken broth
- ♦ 4 teaspoons lemon juice, divided
- ♦ 6 cups chopped romaine lettuce
- ♦ ½ cucumber
- ♦ 1 medium avocado
- ♦ 1 teaspoon fresh dill, chopped
- ♦ 2 teaspoons fresh mint, chopped

METHOD:

1. Over a medium heat, heat the oil in a large pan and then add the lamb.
2. Ensuring that you stir often, cook for 3 minutes before adding the onion.
3. Ensure the lamb is cooked through and the onion has softened.
4. Then stir in the 2 teaspoons lemon juice, chicken broth, thyme and oregano.
5. Add salt and pepper to season. Simmer for a further 5 minutes.
6. While it simmers, you can grate the cucumber and then spread it out on a clean towel before wringing out the excess moisture.
7. Put the grated cucumber in a blender and add 2 teaspoons lemon juice, the avocado, mint, dill and a pinch of salt. Blend until smooth.
8. Serve the meat over chopped lettuce with a spoonful of the delicious avo-tzatziki.

DAY 12 NET CARBS – 11G

Well, well, well. What a day you've got lined up. If you're somehow still feeling peckish, not to worry, you've not even used half of your carb intake for the day.

Breakfast: Pepper Jack Sausage Egg Muffins (See page 32)

Lunch: BALT Wraps (See page 39)

Dinner: Rosemary Lamb Chops

ROSEMARY LAMB CHOPS

Nutrition:

Net carbs – 3g
Protein – 50.5g
Fat – 52g
Calories – 685

INGREDIENTS (FOR 2 SERVINGS):

- 1 tablespoon coconut oil, melted
- 1 teaspoon fresh chopped rosemary
- 1 clove garlic, minced
- 2 bone-in lamb chops (about 150g meat)
- 1 tablespoon butter
- Salt and pepper
- 112.5g fresh asparagus, trimmed
- 1 tablespoon olive oil

METHOD:

1. Syndicate the rosemary, coconut oil, and garlic in a bowl.
2. As you add the lamb chops, coat them in the oil, garlic and rosemary before letting it marinate in the fridge overnight.
3. Before cooking, remove the lamb from the fridge for 30 minutes.
4. Heat the butter in a large pan over medium-high heat.
5. Add the lamb chops and cook for 6 minutes.
6. Season with salt and pepper.
7. Turn the chops over and cook to your desired level.
8. Allow the lamb chops rest away from the heat for 5 minutes before serving.
9. Meanwhile, mix the asparagus with olive oil, salt and pepper. After, spread on a baking sheet.
10. Broil for 6 to 8 minutes until well-cooked. Shake occasionally, and then serve hot with the lamb chops.

DAY 13 NET CARBS – 22.5G

Ever considered filling the gap vacated by the avocado stone? Well, consider it. It provides the perfect space to nestle a fried egg in there. Thank you, mother nature.

Breakfast: Baked Eggs in Avocado

Lunch: Peanut Butter Chicken Thighs (See page 47)

Dinner: Beef Biltong Chilli-Con-Carne (See page 61)

BAKED EGGS IN AVOCADO

Nutrition:

Net carbs – 4.5g
Protein – 20g
Fat – 54g
Calories – 610

INGREDIENTS (1 SERVING):
- 1 medium avocado
- 2 tablespoons lime juice
- 2 tablespoons shredded cheddar cheese
- 2 large eggs
- Salt and pepper

METHOD:

1 Preheat the oven to 225°c and cut the avocado in half.
2 Remove some of the flesh from the middle of each avocado half. And then eat it because Avocado is great.
3 Ensure the avocado halves are upright in the baking dish. Add some lime juice.
4 Crack an egg into each avocado. Season with salt and pepper.
5 Bake for 10 minutes.
6 Sprinkle cheese on top and bake for a few more minutes until the cheese is melted. Serve hot.

DAY 14 NET CARBS – 13G

If you started Day 1 on Monday, that should bring us nicely to a Sunday, the day of the Roast Dinner. And if it isn't Sunday? Well, why not have a Roast in midweek?

Breakfast: Cinnamon Crunch CEREAL (See page 36)

Lunch: Protein-packed Pesto Salad (See page 49)

Dinner: The Rosemary Roast

THE ROSEMARY ROAST

Nutrition:

Net carbs – 8.5g
Protein – 33g
Fat – 40.5
Calories – 540

INGREDIENTS (FOR 2 SERVINGS):

♦ 4 deboned chicken thighs
♦ 2 small carrots, peeled and sliced
♦ 1 small parsnip, peeled and sliced
♦ Salt and pepper
♦ 1 small aubergine, sliced
♦ 1 tablespoon balsamic vinegar
♦ 2 teaspoons fresh chopped rosemary
♦ 2 cloves garlic, sliced
♦ 3 tablespoons olive oil

METHOD:

1. Preheat the oven to 175°c and lightly grease a small rimmed baking sheet with cooking spray.
2. Put the chicken thighs on a baking sheet and add salt and pepper.
3. Arrange the vegetables around the chicken. Get artistic with it if you like. Then sprinkle some sliced garlic.
4. Whisk the remaining ingredients together before drizzling over the chicken and veggies.
5. Bake for 30 minutes.
6. Broil for a further 3 to 5 minutes until the skins are crisp.

DAY 15 NET CARBS – 18.5G

It takes skills to cook skillet. Kill it.

Breakfast: Bacon Breakfast Bombs (See page 33)

Lunch: Keto Carbonara (See page 24)

Dinner: Sausage and Mushroom Skillet

SAUSAGE AND MUSHROOM SKILLET

Nutrition:

Net carbs – 9g
Protein – 33g
Fat – 48g
Calories – 630

INGREDIENTS (FOR 2 SERVINGS):

♦ 1 tablespoon coconut oil
♦ ½ teaspoon dried oregano
♦ ¼ teaspoon dried thyme
♦ ¼ cup marinara sauce
♦ ¼ cup water
♦ ½ cup shredded mozzarella cheese
♦ 150g Italian sausage, crumbled
♦ 150g sliced mushrooms
♦ 1 small yellow onion, chopped
♦ Salt and pepper

METHOD:

1   Preheat the oven to 175c.
2   Heat the oil in large cast-iron pan over medium heat until smoking.
3   Add the sausages and cook until they turn brown and are almost cooked all the way through.
4   Remove the sausages from the pan, and allow them to cool on a cutting board for a few minutes.
5   Add the mushroom and onion to the pan and cook for 3 to 4 minutes until browned.
6   Cut the sausages how you like and add them back to the pan.
7   Mix in the thyme, oregano, salt and pepper.
8   Pour over the sauce and water then stir it all well and truly. Put the pan in the oven and cook for 10 minutes.
9   Sprinkle the mozzarella on top and then cook for another 5 minutes until it's melted.

DAY 16 NET CARBS – 11.5G

It's pizza day. I'm happy for you. Truly. Oh, and don't hold back on the cheese.

Breakfast: Creamy Cheese Omelette (See page 85)

Lunch: Spring Salad with Steak and Sweet Dressing (See page 96)

Dinner: Pan-fried Pepperoni Pizzas

PAN-FRIED PEPPERONI PIZZAS

Nutrition:

Net carbs – 4.5g
Protein – 32g
Fat – 42g
Calories – 545

INGREDIENTS (FOR 3 PIZZAS):

- ◆ 6 large eggs
- ◆ 6 tablespoons grated parmesan cheese
- ◆ 3 tablespoons psyllium husk powder
- ◆ 1 ½ teaspoons Italian seasoning
- ◆ 3 tablespoons olive oil
- ◆ 9 tablespoons low-carb tomato sauce, divided
- ◆ 112.5g shredded mozzarella, divided
- ◆ 112.5 g diced pepperoni, divided
- ◆ 3 tablespoons fresh chopped basil

METHOD:

1 Combine the psyllium husk powder, eggs and parmesan with the Italian seasoning and a pinch of salt in a blender.
2 Blend for about 30 seconds until smooth, then set it aside for 5 minutes.
3 Heat 1 tablespoon of oil in a pan over medium-high heat.
4 Spoon 1/3 of the batter into the pan and spread in a circle then cook until browned underneath.
5 Turn the pizza crust over and cook until browned on the other side.
6 Remove the crust to a foil-lined baking sheet before repeating with the batter that remains.
7 Scoop 3 tablespoons of low-carb tomato sauce over each crust.
8 Top with diced pepperoni and shredded cheese before boiling until the cheese is browned.
9 Sprinkle with fresh basil before slicing the pizza to serve.

DAY 17 NET CARBS – 19.5G

Scrambled eggs to start, Melting cheesy tuna for lunch, creamy, delicious, healthy, wonderful Risotto for dinner.

Breakfast: Veggie Scrambled Eggs (See page 30)

Lunch: Mozzarella Tuna Melt

Dinner: Mushroom Cauliflower Rice Risotto (See page 20)

MOZZARELLA TUNA MELT

Nutrition:

Net carbs – 10.5g
Protein – 45g
Fat – 36g
Calories – 550

INGREDIENTS (FOR 2 SERVINGS):

- 200g canned tuna
- ½ cup diced yellow onion
- 1 tablespoon olive oil
- 2 large eggs, whisked
- 50g shredded mozzarella cheese
- ¼ cup mayonnaise
- Salt and pepper
- 1 green onion, sliced thin

METHOD:

1. In a pan over medium heat, heat the oil.
2. Add the onion and cook for about 5 minutes until it starts to become transparent.
3. Drain the tuna and then put it into the pan and mix in the ingredients that remain.
4. Add salt and pepper and cook for 2 minutes until the cheese melts.
5. Scoop the contents into a bowl before topping with the sliced onion to serve.

DAY 18 NET CARBS – 11.5G

Sumptuous chicken thighs after an oh-so wholesome morning.

Breakfast: The Keto Fry-up (See page 34)

Lunch: Gyro Salad with Avo-Tzatziki (See page 87)

Dinner: Crispy Chipotle Chicken Thighs

CRISPY CHIPOTLE CHICKEN THIGHS

Nutrition:

Net carbs – 1.5
Protein – 51g
Fat – 20g
Calories – 400

INGREDIENTS (FOR 2 SERVINGS):

- ♦ ½ teaspoon chipotle chili powder
- ♦ ¼ teaspoon smoked paprika
- ♦ ¼ teaspoon garlic powder
- ♦ ¼ teaspoon onion powder
- ♦ ¼ teaspoon ground coriander
- ♦ 300g boneless chicken thighs
- ♦ Salt and pepper
- ♦ 1 tablespoon olive oil
- ♦ 3 cups fresh baby spinach

METHOD:

1. Combine the smoked paprika, garlic powder, onion powder, coriander and chipotle chili powder, in a bowl.
2. Pound the chicken thighs until they are flat. Season with salt and pepper on both sides and then cut them in half.
3. Heat the oil in a pan over medium-high heat.
4. Add the chicken thighs to the pan skin-side-down and sprinkle the spice mixture over them.
5. Cook the chicken thighs for 8 minutes before flipping and cooking them on the other side for 3 to 5 minutes. During the last 3 minutes, add the spinach to the pan and cook until soft and wilted.
6. Serve the crispy chicken thighs on top of the spinach.

DAY 19 NET CARBS – 21G

Zoodle. What on earth is zoodle? Zebra noodles? Zen noodles? Not even noodles at all? Well, you're about to find out.

Breakfast: Sweet Blueberry Coconut Porridge (See page 70)

Lunch: Bouyiourdi (See page 51)

Dinner: Chicken Zoodle Alfredo

CHICKEN ZOODLE ALFREDO

Nutrition:

Net carbs – 3g
Protein – 55g
Fat – 40g
Calories – 595

INGREDIENTS (FOR 2 SERVINGS):

- ♦ 2 (200g) chicken breasts
- ♦ ¼ cup grated parmesan cheese
- ♦ 200g courgette
- ♦ 1 tablespoon olive oil
- ♦ Salt and pepper
- ♦ 2 tablespoons butter
- ♦ ¼ cup heavy cream

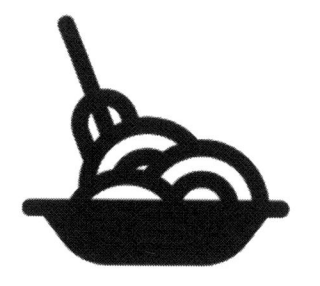

METHOD:

1 In a large pan, heat the oil over a medium-high heat.
2 Season the chicken with salt and pepper before adding to the pan.
3 Cook for 6 to 7 minutes on each side until cooked through.
4 Remove the chicken from the pan and slice it into strips.
5 Reheat the pan over medium-low heat and add the butter.
6 Mix in the heavy cream and parmesan cheese then cook until it is nice and thick.
7 Twist the courgette into fancy little spirals and then toss it into the sauce mixture with the chicken.
8 Cook the courgette for about 2 minutes until it is tender and then serve hot.

DAY 20 NET CARBS – 23.5G

Keeping it oriental with this fried egg mushroom soup. It's delicious and light leaving plenty of room for your keto carbonara in the evening. And as for breakfast, well, that speaks for itself.

Breakfast: Bacon Breakfast Bombs (See page 33)

Lunch: Fried Egg Mushroom Soup

Dinner: Keto Shepherd's Pie (See page 65)

FRIED EGG MUSHROOM SOUP

Nutrition:

Net carbs – 7g
Protein – 20g
Fat – 31g
Calories – 385

INGREDIENTS (FOR 2 SERVINGS):

- ◆ 3 tablespoons heavy cream
- ◆ 2 tablespoons shredded cheese
- ◆ 1 teaspoon olive oil
- ◆ 1 teaspoon butter
- ◆ 100g riced cauliflower
- ◆ 1 large egg
- ◆ 4 white mushrooms, sliced thin
- ◆ 1 cup vegetable broth

METHOD:

1. Prepare some cauliflower rice, which you should be an expert at by now. If not, go back to the keto basics and learn how to make it.
2. In a small saucepan over medium heat, heat the oil.
3. Then put the mushrooms in and cook for about 6 minutes until they are tender.
4. Mix in the vegetable broth, cauliflower rice and heavy cream.
5. Add salt and pepper before mixing in the cheese.
6. Make the soup as thick as you like it by simmering it, and when it's how you desire, remove from heat.
7. Fry the egg in the butter to a level that you like and then serve it over the soup.

DAY 21 NET CARBS – 15.5G

Lasagne. For those lovers of this layered food, I am sorry that we have made you wait until the very end to reveal this absolute diamond to you. Courgette plays the role of the sheets in this oh so delicious end to 21-day keto diet plan. You should now be firing with your keto lifestyle and equipped with an array of low-carb meals that will blow people's minds.

Breakfast: Cinnamon Crunch CEREAL (See page 36)
Lunch: Ham and Cheese Waffles (See page 42)
Dinner: Cheesy Courgette Lasagne

CHEESY COURGETTE LASAGNE

Nutrition:

Net carbs – 8.5g
Protein – 29g
Fat – 19g
Calories – 325

INGREDIENTS (FOR 1 LASAGNA):
♦ 75g shredded mozzarella
♦ 1 small courgette (60g), sliced very thin into rounds
♦ 2 tablespoons ricotta cheese
♦ 3 tablespoons low-carb marinara sauce
♦ Dried oregano

METHOD:

1. Spoon a tablespoon of the marinara sauce into a microwavable bowl.
2. Place one third of the courgette slices on top of the sauce and then add a tablespoon of ricotta on top of the slices.
3. Repeat this process to create more layers. Sauce, courgette, and ricotta.
4. Place any remaining courgette on top and add the last tablespoon of marinara.
5. Sprinkle with mozzarella on top and then microwave for 3 to 4 minutes. When removing, ensure that the entire mixture is heated through and that the cheese is melted.
6. Garnish with dried oregano and serve hot.

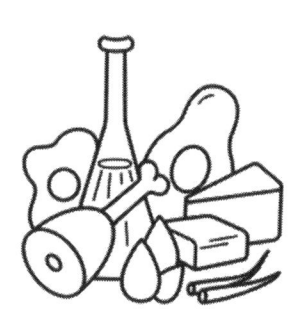

DISCLAIMER

This book contains opinions and ideas of the author and is meant to teach the reader informative and helpful knowledge while due care should be taken by the user in the application of the information provided. The instructions and strategies are possibly not right for every reader and there is no guarantee that they work for everyone. Using this book and implementing the information/recipes therein contained is explicitly your own responsibility and risk. This work with all its contents, does not guarantee correctness, completion, quality or correctness of the provided information. Misinformation or misprints cannot be completely eliminated.